DIVINING ECSTASY
THE MAGICAL & MYSTICAL
ESSENCE OF
SALVIA DIVINORUM

DIVINING ECSTASY
THE MAGICAL & MYSTICAL ESSENCE OF SALVIA DIVINORUM

by Dr. Sean Shayan

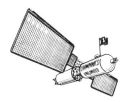

Loompanics Unlimited
Port Townsend, Washngton

Neither the author nor the publisher assumes any responsibility for the use or misuse of information contained in this book. It is sold for entertainment purposes only. Be warned!

Published by:
Loompanics Unlimited
PO Box 1197
Port Townsend, WA 98368
Loompanics Unlimited is a division of Loompanics Enterprises, Inc.
Phone: 360-385-2230
E-mail: service@loompanics.com
Web site: www.loompanics.com

Cover by Dr. Sean Shayan
Salvia Divinorum photos courtesy of Botanic-Art, Netherlands
    and Sean Shayan
Illustrations by J. Blanchard

ISBN 1-55950-221-5
Library of Congress Card Catalog Number 2001093173

Contents

For Asa

WARNING: *Some medicinal and psychoactive plants may be harmful to your health. Some are more dangerous than others. Some are safer than others. Each person will react differently to each substance. Readers are advised to consult with a medical professional prior to ingesting any plant or psychoactive substance. Further, readers are advised that they use such substances entirely at their own risk. The author and the publisher of this book disclaim any and all liability for any adverse effects, including but not limited to death resulting from the use of any plant or other substance that is discussed herein.*

Salvia and Drug Testing

Salvia cannot be detected by any current drug tests. It is unlikely that a test can or will be developed for this. Since little or no known testing has been done on this, the current detection period for *Salvia divinorum* metabolites in urine is unknown. *Salvia divinorum* is not an illegal plant and its metabolites are not restricted as of the publishing of this book. The presence of *Salvia divinorum* metabolites should not be of any concern even if testing is possible; however driving or operation of heavy machinery while intoxicated on *any* mind altering substance is illegal. There are incidences of people being charged with DUI (Driving Under the Influence) when all they had taken was Kava Kava or other common health foods or other nonscheduled substances. Needless to say common sense should dictate that one does not drive or operate heavy machinery while under the influence of a strong psychotropic substance such as *Salvia divinorum*.

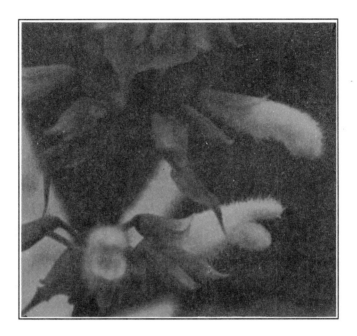

Salvia divinorum

Introduction

As more and more people around the world are opening their hearts and minds to access inner, spiritual knowledge, they are coming to understand the profound benefits that can be obtained through the use of psychedelic substances. Ethnobotany is the study of how different indigenous cultures utilize plants for food, shelter, medicine and religious ceremonies. Today ethnobotanists study these cultures and their use of plants, distilling their herbal wisdom for the benefit of those who live in technologically advanced societies.

With the progress of medical technology, natural remedies have been brushed aside in favor of chemically produced medicines. But the tide is turning; both consumers and medical experts are beginning to look back to the origins of medicine and the possible therapeutic effects of plants.

Plants have always been used in medicine, and are found in many of the commonly used pharmaceuticals today. Now with increasing numbers of socially conscious people looking for alternatives to the western medicines that are often detrimental to the human organism, plant therapy is re-emerging as the wave of the future.

However, the scourge of genetic engineering and the destruction of the rainforests and other natural resources present alarming obstacles. Not only are we tampering with the ecological systems that have kept us alive for millions of years, but we are also rapidly depleting the stock of indigenous plants that could provide the cure for many diseases. The destruction of the rainforest also threatens to destroy the indigenous people whose knowledge of the plants and how to use them to their full potential could prove invaluable.

Salvia divinorum, a species of sage from the mint family (*labiatae*), is a plant native to Oaxaca, Mexico. Otherwise known as the "Diviner's Sage," it can be used both as a curative and as an aid to attaining epic, mind-altering states. The shamans of the Mazatec Indian villages have used this plant primarily in divination and healing.

Although the Mazatecs have used this plant for at least five hundred years, knowledge of it in the West began in the 1950s. An early report by Roberto Weitlaner recorded the use of *hierba de Maria* (leaf or herb of Mary) in a curing ritual in the small Oaxacan village of Jalapa de Diaz. A sample of this herb was later sent to Dr. Carl Epling who identified and named the plant *Salvia divinorum*.

The Mazatecs regard the plant as holy and take special care not to trample or destroy the plant when they cut it from the wild, even kneeling to pray to it before they take it. Many Mazatecan curanderos (shamans) believe that the plant is an incarnation of the Virgin Mary as a Shepherdess, and call the plant *ska Maria Pastora*. These indigenous initiates use the plant to induce prophetic vision. They are also very protective of its growing place and will not show any outsiders where it hides.

There have been only rare sightings of this plant growing wild. All information about *salvia divinorum* has been gleaned from clones, cuttings and specimens of the plant retrieved by the Mazatecs. Perhaps they conceal it for good reason: this is not a plant to be trifled with. It must be regarded with the proper respect for its lessons to be imparted to the reverent user.

By studying these cultures and their healing plants, we may discover that the importance of these plant species goes far beyond ancient "folk remedies." Exploration of its potential can only yield positive results as we seek to find *Salvia*'s place in the pantheon of ethnobotanical gods and healers.

Chapter One
Present and Past

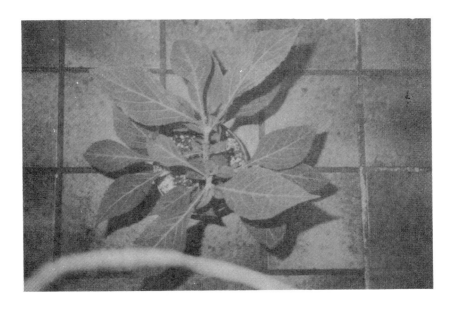

It is night and two men and a woman sit in a darkened room talking quietly, faces illuminated only by the light licking at them from the candles on the table. They are preparing to ingest the plant *Salvia divinorum,* and embark on a journey in consciousness. The plant and its effects are not widely known throughout the United States and Europe although it is becoming better known now than ever before in history. Its newly-found recognition is due, in the main, to the rise of the Internet and the availability of such information to the masses.

Until recently, *Salvia divinorum* has been known only to the native people who traditionally have employed the plant in their religious ceremonies — the indigenous people of Oaxaca, Mexico, the Mazatec Indians. But with the help of a few curious psychonauts and a handful of scientists interested in the psychoactive and healing effects of certain plant materials, *Salvia* has found her way into the hands of certain responsible parties intrigued by the possibility of being taught by this plant guide.

The people gathered in the room are prepared for such a lesson. The female decides to go first. She empties the dried leaves that have been treated with a 5x extract of the active principle in *Salvia, Salvinorin A*, into a medium-sized pipe bowl attached to a small glass bong. After lighting the material, she pulls steadily on the bong until the smoke reaches her lips and is thickly filled in the glass tube and then she releases the bowl from its cradle and inhales the spirit of the plant.

(5x extract means 5 grams of leaf were extracted to make 1 gram of extract, hence 5x. This means that one gram of a 5x extract is equal in strength to 5 grams of leaf. Salvia comes in varying strengths and potencies. The most common are 5x, 6x, and 10x extracts. However, the 10x extracts which we tested seemed in many cases to be the equivalent of the 6x extracts currently on the market. The author suggests using a 6x extract. The best on the market is the Divination brand Salvia Divinorum extract offered by Temple of Ecstacy Corporation — see Resources. Making your own extract is not recommended as it is messy and not worth the hassle unless you are an expert in extraction and have all of the necessary equipment. Fine quality extracts are readily available and easy to obtain.)

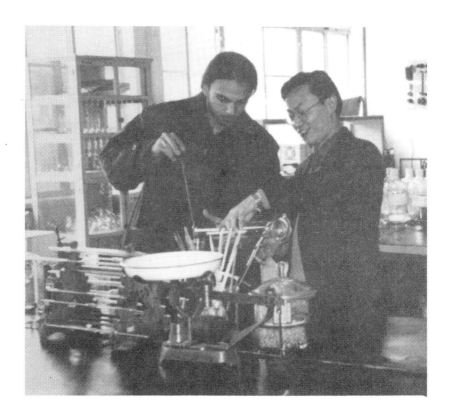

Obviously, this method is not the one favored by the Mazatecs in their shamanic rituals of healing. They would take the fresh leaves of the plant and grind them against a stone metate to express the liquid essence from the herb. This is then strained through a sieve, passed through copal incense and drunk reverently, all part of an elaborate divination ritual. Or, alternatively, they roll bundles of the fresh leaves into a quid, which is then chewed for up to half an hour, allowing the liquid essence of the leaves to permeate the mouth cavity. For a long time people in the Western world believed that the only way to produce the active effects was through the grinding of fresh leaves and that the active ingredient was rendered inactive upon drying. The active principle is thought to be absorbed through the oral mucosa. Therefore, either chewing the leaves and holding the liquid in one's mouth, or else grinding the leaves to produce a liquid to be drunk, were the only ways thought possible to experience *Salvia*'s world.

Further research proved this to be untrue. Today it is recognized that dried *Salvia* leaves, when smoked from a water pipe or bong, can produce the visionary effects known to the Mazatecs. Although smoking may produce effects of a shorter duration and less intense nature than an abundance of chewed material, there is sufficient evidence to indicate that the active principle does, in fact, remain in the dried leaves. However, to get the total effect from smoking, it is necessary to inhale large amounts of the smoke and it must be smoked using a water pipe of some sort because *Salvia* requires large amounts of heat to vaporize appropriately.

The woman exhales the smoke slowly, holding in her breath as long as possible. Her two male companions watch with interest. Until that point they had only read of *Salvia*'s effects. Many Internet pages are devoted to "trip reports" on various substances, including *Salvia divinorum*, and the reports seem unique to each experience.

All three were curious to discover how *Salvia* might approach them. After all of the smoke is exhaled from her lungs, the woman sits back on the floor and looks at her two friends. She reports that she isn't feeling anything yet but smiles as she says this. They tell her to give it a little time. Within a few minutes, she decides to take another small hit to see if it will initiate the experience. After taking the second hit, she begins to laugh a bit shakily, and nods her head to indicate that the effects are beginning to take hold. She lies back for a minute or so, flat on the ground but with her hands in the air as if seeing something there and trying to grasp it. Almost immediately she rises again with her eyes open and begins talking to the men, trying to explain what she is seeing, but becomes disoriented and loses track of what she is saying.

The men look at each other with grins, and tell the girl not to worry, that it is okay if she can't tell them what is going on. She seems slightly irritated and confused and looks at them blankly.

All literature on *Salvia* will explain the importance of having a sitter while experimenting with this potent hallucinogen. Even in the Mazatec culture it is common for a sober person to watch over the ceremony to ensure that all participants are free from harm. Especially with personal psychonautic journeys, it is imperative to have someone present to help navigate the way in case one becomes lost. If the experience becomes frightening, too intense or disorienting for the voyager, the guide can reassure him or her that all is well and that the experience will soon pass. The guide can also ensure the participant's physical safety by keeping him or her from wandering outside, attempting to drive a car or causing any harm to their person or home.

The *Salvia* experience can be so intense that participants may actually lose track of their bodies, and though seemingly aware and conscious of their actions are, in truth, only using their bodies as a vehicle to maneuver through the unfamiliar world in which their brains are functioning. It is as if body and mind are separate and the voyager is unaware of the physical reality that is actually surrounding his or her body. This is why having someone sober to observe and enforce physical boundaries is always a prudent idea.

The initial, intense effects of smoked *Salvia* usually only last from five to fifteen minutes with an almost complete return to a normal mental state within half an hour, although lingering effects may pervade the body for up to an hour and a half. The lingering effects are mostly feelings of relaxation, calm, and clarity, although some lightheadedness and slight disorientation may occur.

After a few minutes of struggling to communicate with her companions, the woman's face takes on a more relaxed posture and she smiles again, explaining that she knows what is going on now. She remembers smoking the drug and she lies back down on the floor with her eyes shut for the remainder of the trip. Within ten minutes she is sitting up again, talking to her friends, trying to explain what she saw and asking them what, if anything, she had said. She doesn't remember the first few minutes of the trip. She then says that she felt as though she were surrounded by people that had been at the house earlier that night, and they were asking her questions, which she was struggling to answer. This is when she remembers feeling disoriented and reports feeling like she wanted to cry because she couldn't explain what was going on and felt as if she were under interrogation.

However, she reports that as soon as the guys began to tell her it would be all right in a little while, she remembered that she had smoked the plant.

"It was as if I didn't know where I was or how I got there and yet I had always been there and felt like I might always be. When reality began to creep back into my consciousness, I realized that I had just smoked a strange substance and lay back down to finish the ride."

This sense of disembodiment and disorientation of time and space is not unusual in the use of *Salvia*. Perhaps it is this very effect that made it useful in shamanic rituals, allowing the shamans to travel outside of their bodies and contact the "other world" that exists coincident with our own.

Plant hallucinogens have been used since the beginning of civilization, in almost all native cultures, as a means for accessing the spirit world and accessing the healing properties of the gods that reside in the plants. The native peoples understood the idea that all living things possess a spirit and it is with this belief that they pray to the plant gods and invoke their strength while ingesting the magic herbs, vines or fungi.

After the woman is done with her "journey," the men are anxious to try it. They know they have nothing to be afraid of. They have watched its effects with their own eyes, and although their friend had become slightly agitated, the discomfort was of short duration. The smaller man decides to go first, wrongly assuming they could then determine the amount needed to get the larger man off based on body size.

Salvia does not work this way. It is uniquely individual in that certain people are naturally more sensitive to the effects and may need very little to produce profound effects. Conversely, there are some people who seem impervious to the drug's effects and can consume great quantities without ever leaving their comfortable realities for the unknown realms of this plant goddess.

The smaller man proves this by taking three enormous hits from the same bong as his friend, but describes only a vague sense of floating and attendant lightheadedness. The woman had reported a definite sense of her body sinking into the ground and her consciousness being somewhere else. The smaller man shakes his head in bewilderment and says he doesn't feel much different. The larger man takes the bong and tries for himself, using almost the same quantity as the woman, but less than his smaller counterpart.

As soon as he exhales the first hit, he takes some deep breaths and immediately fills the bowl and takes another. Before he can even put the bong and lighter down he begins to laugh. He then closes his eyes and lies back on the floor.

His companions watch as his feet and legs move occasionally as if he were swimming or floating, propelling himself through water. He continues to smile throughout the trip but says nothing. After about fifteen minutes, he sits up and describes his journey:

"I didn't have the visuals that K. did, although there was a white light that seemed to pervade through my sight and then sort of reached down through me splitting me apart leaving trails of red and green light behind. I felt as if I were kind of floating on this river of light and I could feel the light moving through me."

He says his experience was very pleasant and he had no feelings of anxiety or detachment from reality, but more of a deep relaxation. Afterward he was quite calm and wanted to turn on some music saying he felt very peaceful and still somewhat intoxicated, though not in the way that one is intoxicated with alcohol or Cannabis, more like "being intoxicated with life or religion."

Chapter Two
History of Our Lady,
Ska Maria Pastora

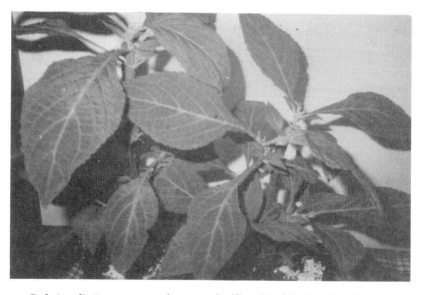

Salvia divinorum — it sounds like Buddha's drool, but actually, this little plant is a powerful entheogen traditionally used by the Mazatec Indians as a tool in curing and divination. A rare Mexican sage, she has been used for many years in the indigenous culture of the Sierra Mazateca and grows in the outer forest ravines of this area. *Salvia* is an elusive plant; wild specimens are difficult to find and aside from the reports from A. Reisfield telling of various populations growing through the Sierra Mazateca in 1985, no other sightings have been made and some scientists doubt that it grows wild anymore. Many scientists now believe that it may always have been a cultigen. All information about this sage has been gleaned from clones, and most from the original specimen sent to the states by famous entheogen researchers, Gordon Wasson and Albert Hofmann.

Wasson was the first white man to journey to the Sierra Mazateca in search of information about the Mexican mushroom cults. He was aware that these entheogenic fungi were used in shamanic ceremonies and divination rituals. During his research, his attention was alerted to the growth and use of another plant, *hojas de la Pastora* or *ska Maria Pastora*, the leaves of Mary the Shepherdess, our *Salvia divinorum*. During his time in Ayautla, Wasson requested the leaves instead of the mushrooms for a divination rite performed by curandera Augustina Borja. Wasson drank the liquid that had been squeezed from the leaves and noted what each participant from then on would: it is bitter indeed.

Wasson describes his first experience:

"The effect of the leaves came sooner than would have been the case with mushrooms, was less sweeping, and lasted a shorter time. There was not the slightest doubt about the effect, but it did not go beyond the initial effect of the mushrooms, i.e., dancing colors in elaborate, three-dimensional designs. Whether a larger dose would have produced a greater effect, I do not know."[1]

---

[1] Wasson, R. Gordon. (1962). "A New Mexican Psychotropic Drug from the Mint Family," Harvard University Botanical Museum Leaflets, obtained through Erowid.org.

After completing his research with the mushrooms, Wasson decided to investigate this new plant further and called on his old friend, Albert Hofmann. Together with Hofmann's wife, Anita, and Irmgard Weitlaner Johnson, (whose father Robert Weitlaner and former husband Jean B. Johnson, had contributed greatly to the study of the Mexican mushrooms), he traveled back to the beautiful Sierra Mazateca in search of this new plant goddess.

Before their journey in the fall of 1962, little had been heard of this sage. It could be that the Mexicans realized its worth and said nothing of it to outsiders. They take great care in hiding its growing place and treat the plant with great respect, as they do with all sacred items. It could also be that because *Salvia* has a more subtle power than the magic mushrooms, discussion of its potential was eclipsed by the other entheogen. However, there are some historical mentions. Robert Weitlaner mentions the use of the *hierba de Maria* in a curing ritual in the small Oaxacan village of Jalapa de Diaz. And the descriptions found of the Aztec plant, pipiltzintzintli, seem to fit *Salvia*, although more scientists now believe the reports refer to *Cannabis sativa*. So, Wasson and Hofmann would be the first to travel specifically to find, identify and work with la dame *Salvia*.

In Chapter Six of his book, *LSD: My Problem Child*, Hofmann describes their trek to Oaxaca in search of *ska Maria Pastora* and the difficulty they encountered in finding a shaman or curandera to bring them to the plant and to perform the sacred ceremonies for them. Dona Herlinda, who would act as their interpreter while in Mazatec country, had become a friend of Wasson's during his previous journeys through the region. She would prove to be a powerful liaison between the scientists and the native peoples and their plant secrets.

"The desired contact with persons skilled in medicine came about thanks to the kindred connections of Dona Herlinda, beginning with the curandero Don Sabino. But he refused, for some reason, to receive us in a consultation and to question the leaves.

"From an old curandera, a venerable woman in a strikingly magnificent Mazatec garment, with the lovely name Natividad Rosa, we received a whole bundle of flowering specimens of the sought after plant. But even she could not be prevailed upon to perform a ceremony with the leaves, nor would Natividad Rosa tell us where she had gathered the leaves. They grew in a very, very distant forest valley. Wherever she dug up a plant, she put a coffee bean in the earth as a thanks to the gods."[2]

It isn't easy for researchers and scientists to ingratiate themselves with the indigenous people of cultures like the Mazatecs. These people hold their sacred ceremonies close to them and are mostly unwilling to share the information with Westerners who may desecrate what they make holy. The curanderas (and curanderos) also fear that their powers may fall into the hands of a rival or someone who might use their magic for evil purposes.

A journal article entitled, "The Ethnopharmacology of Ska Maria Pastora," discusses this common problem:

"The jealous and secretive nature of native shamans works against statistical methods of survey. Visiting many shamans in a single area can actually lessen the amount of information gathered, as each curandero may fear the visitor is telling their

---

[2] Hofmann, A. "In Search of the Magic Plant Ska Maria Pastora in the Mazatec Country," *LSD: My Problem Child*, obtained from Lycaeum.org.

secrets and giving their power to a rival. To them magic can hurt or kill."[3]

For Wasson and Hofmann this proved to be a difficulty. It seemed that angry neighbors or colleagues had burned the house of Maria Sabina because she had shown the strangers the magic of the mushrooms. Maria had held the first ceremony for Wasson in his private travels. Hofmann also notes that "the profanation of the mushroom cult did not stop with the scientific investigations. The publication about the magic mushrooms unleashed an invasion of hippies and drug seekers into the Mazatec country, many of whom behaved badly, some even criminally."[4] It is little wonder why the people of this region are protective of their sacred plants and sacred traditions. But in the name of scientific discovery, an understanding and sensitive few must press on.

This is precisely what Wasson and company did. After receiving the first flowering samples from Natividad Rosa, they took the leaves and pressed them in the traditional method for ingestion. Hofmann undertook the task of grinding the leaves under the guidance of a young Indian girl familiar with this method. Believing that the active principle in *Salvia* must be contained in the leaves since this was the only part of the plant that the Mazatecs used, Hofmann took the liquid from the samples, mixed it with alcohol for preservation and decanted it into flasks for later experimentation and study. Although Hofmann did not know this at the time, *Salvia* extract loses its potency after being freshly pressed and the preserved extract would yield no positive results later. This led the scientists to conclude that the active compound was unstable.

---

[3] Valdes, L.J. III, Diaz J.L. and Paul, Ara G. (1983) "Ethnopharmacology of Ska Maria Pastora," *Journal of Ethnopharmacology.*
[4] Hofmann.

Wasson and Hofmann did finally come across a curendera who would perform a ceremony for them. It was done in secret, to avoid any retribution. The curandera, Consuela Garcia, began the ceremony by burning copal resin, sacred incense necessary for the ritual. Consuela then prepared the leaves, counting them out in pairs for each of the participants, which is the traditional way, not only for *Salvia*, but for the magic mushrooms as well. The pairs of leaves represent both the male and female, the balance of nature.

During this first ceremony, Hofmann had to watch, admitting he was not well due to the change in environment. He observed while his wife and Wasson drank from the prepared potion. After about twenty minutes of sitting in the dark, Anita and Wasson both agreed that they could perceive mild effects of the plant in the form of brightly colored images or patterns. As Wasson had noted from his previous experience, the effects were less intense and shorter in duration than the effects of mushrooms, but still possessed a distinctive hallucinogenic quality.

The curandera questioned them about their belief in the holiness of the ceremony. Once this was affirmed, Consuela continued with the ritual, lighting the candles again, placing them under the images of the saints that decorated the altar table and singing and chanting what were either prayers or magical incantations. For the native people these ceremonies are highly religious and inextricable from their beliefs in Christianity and the saints. They employ plants like *Salvia* or mushrooms as a way of reaching out to these invisible entities, making contact, and receiving either healing information or the transfer of power to heal. Sometimes in these ceremonies, only the curandera (or curandero) will drink of the potion and use the ceremony to divine the problem. More often, both the curandera (or curandero) and the patient will take the drink and collaborate on the healing process.

A few days after this initial experiment, Hofmann himself was able to try *Salvia* while the rest of the company took pills of psilocybin in a mushroom ceremony with the famous curandera, Maria Sabina. Sabina was interested in the little pills, which contained the "spirit" of the mushrooms: about 5mg of psilocybin. It is hard for native people to understand the scientific method of extraction and isolation of active principles of plants, and because of this Sabina was skeptical that the pills could be as effective as the sacred mushrooms.

While the others indulged in the psilocybin pills, five pairs of fresh *Salvia* leaves were prepared ceremoniously for Hofmann. The curanderas and the others experienced high levels of inebriation, accompanied by the euphoria and mystical visions typical with the mushroom ceremony. Hofmann reported that he found himself "in a state of mental sensitivity and intense experience" but that it wasn't "accompanied by hallucinations."

So this first foray into the Mazatec in search of *hierba de la Pastora* was both successful and unsuccessful. Wasson and Hofmann were able to procure samples for identification, which were studied and named by Dr. Carl Epling as *Salvia divinorum.* They were able to confirm that the plant was used as a substitute for the mushrooms in native ceremonies and thus concluded that the effects of the plant must be along the same psychoactive lines as the psilocybin in mushrooms. However, they were not able to experience the intensity level they expected or hoped for while using the plant. And they were unable to preserve the juice for later chemical analysis, only proving that whatever active principle the plant contained, it was highly unstable and, therefore, probably not of the same physical make-up of other known hallucinogens. The doorway to this magical plant was merely revealed, with no answer to the question of what might lie beyond that door.

Leander J. Valdes, Jose Luis Diaz, and Ara G. Paul documented other experiments and commented on the traditions of Mazatec healing in their previously mentioned journal article, "The Ethnopharmacology of Ska Maria Pastora." They investigated this plant after curiosity had been aroused by accounts of its use from Wasson and Hofmann. The active principle had yet to be determined but this group of scientists set out to learn more about the reputed ability of *Salvia* to induce prophetic visions.

Their main guide and source for information regarding the sacred herb was Don Alejandro. He explained to them the nature of the plant and its use as a healer in shamanic rituals, as well as performing a divination ceremony for them. Because of their association with a university and Don Alejandro's belief that the experiments and information were being given away in the interest of science to promote a greater understanding of *Salvia* as curative, he did not fear imparting his wisdom to the "Westerners" as did other shamans before him.

Don Alejandro told them of the integral part that *Salvia* plays in the initiation of a young curandero apprentice on the path to healing. Over the course of about two years, a typical duration for shaman apprenticeship, the initiate uses different hallucinogenic plants to facilitate communication with the gods and to learn the art of healing from them. There are three levels to reach, and since *Salvia* is the mildest, she is the natural starting point. After mastery of her lessons, the initiate gradually moves on to the morning glory seeds (which contain lysergic acid amide) and then finally to the sacred mushrooms.

Although (when chewed) the psychotropic effects of *Salvia divinorum* are not as strong as the effects of the sacred mushrooms, which many practiced shamans prefer to use in their ceremonies, the *Salvia* plant is important to the Mazatecs for a different reason: she is perceived as an unparalleled healer. The Mazatecs believe that the plant is the incarnation of the Virgin Mary, hence the name *ska Maria Pastora. Salvia* has many names but they all refer to this sacred connection. It is interesting to note that the Mazatecs didn't seem to have a native name for the plant until after the conquest by the Spanish, from whom they derived their Christian beliefs. But they are nominal Christians, incorporating the gods and saints of Christianity into their own native practices and ceremonies. *Ska Maria Pastora* is the first to be used in the shaman's journey on the "way to heaven" because the Virgin Mary is said to be the best teacher of the gods. She is able to instruct the young curanderos in the ways of healing through herbs and plants. Religion and healing are inextricable from each other in most native cultures, a concept far removed from Western medicine, but one that shouldn't be simply dismissed.

During a ceremony performed for both Diaz and Valdes, in which they participated along with Don Alejandro while Don Alejandro's son kept watch, the scientists gained a better understanding of the important role of religion in the ceremony and the sacredness of the rituals in which they were partaking.

After an elaborate prayer, which invoked the power of Jesus and the Saints and asked for sacred guidance from Mary and the gods and for the protection for the subjects (Diaz and Valdes), Don Alejandro administered the *Salvia* infusion to the group. The curandero encouraged Diaz and Valdes to speak, explaining that unless they described their visions they would be unable to learn the lessons being shown to them by the gods. When Don Alejandro became distressed that his two subjects seemed unable to access the "gods," Diaz tried to assure him that it was through no fault of the curandero, or of the plant. He explained that they came from different cultures and were bound to approach the visions from a different perspective. This is an important point related to *Salvia*, because the person and his or her background and perceptions (or, the set and setting) are essential parts of the *Salvia* experience and can color the journey in any number of shades: from shallow light to intense, horrifying dark.

Valdes and Diaz had greater success than previous explorers, Wasson and Hofmann, in achieving more traditional hallucinogenic visions, but they also had consumed leaves in a far greater quantity (about 50-60 pairs of leaves). The effects included visions of both people and objects, although it became apparent that the visions were subject in part to suggestion. When one participant would describe what he was seeing, the other's vision would start to change and incorporate the same imagery. The implications of this aren't well understood, but may be important nevertheless. Could it be that *Salvia* and other hallucinogens give us access to another world where these spirits and objects actually exist and with the right direction we may all be able to see the same alternate reality? Could it be that this world "which is invisible, nearby and far away" is available with the help of this plant goddess as a guide? Or maybe our minds are already susceptible to the power of suggestion and the plant only induces an increased sensitivity in the brain which allows us to experience whatever we wish, including a shared visionary world.

Chapter Three
The Beauty of Salvia

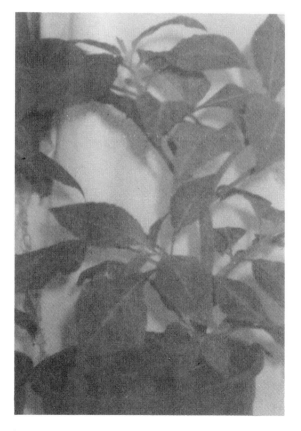

Salvia divinorum is an aesthetic plant that any botaniphile would be happy to grow as a decorative houseplant, even if they had no knowledge of the potent magic it holds within. The perennial plant grows to three feet tall and beyond, if properly supported, and can be easily maintained by an earnest gardener. Once she reaches a certain height, her hollow stem will bend or break and the branches may take root in viable soil. Because *Salvia* rarely seeds from her flower, it is usually propagated by cuttings from healthy plants or from the natural re-growth described above.

Her leaves are oval with serrated edges. They are usually a bright green but can be a light celery color that may appear almost yellow at times. This yellow color may be a sign of too much water, a condition that drains the chlorophyll-producing nutrients that would normally provide the rich green color. To remedy this, a reduction in water is obviously necessary. Adding fertilizer containing chelated iron will also help restore the leaves to their healthy color.

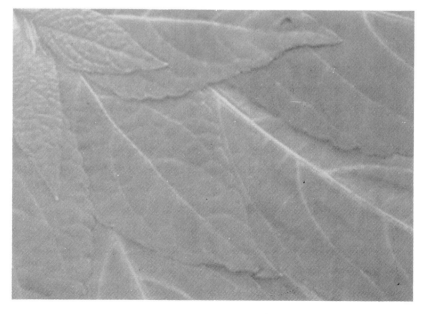

Initially, *Salvia* was mistakenly reported to have blue flowers. We now know that the blue color comes from the calyces out of which a magnificent white corolla blooms. She blooms in late fall and what a beautiful sight that is.

Salvia divinorum was found indigenously in the forest ravines of the Sierra Mazateca, where partial sunlight and humidity were in perfect balance for *Salvia*'s taste. In order to grow *Salvia* one must work to achieve this same balance. The ideal temperature for *Salvia* plants is between 60 and 70 degrees, but plants can survive higher temperatures and drier climates if they get enough water. If you live in a less-than-ideal climate, many gardeners suggest making a humidity tent for the plants to ensure optimum growth. Humidity tents can be purchased from a nursery or through gardening magazines, or they can be constructed using a little ingenuity. People can make a humidity tent by using a regular screen tent typically used by campers to keep the mosquitoes out. Then by setting a humidifier on a timer or by hand-misting a few times a day, you will have created a perfect climate for your plant.

Cultivating a plant through a cutting is the most popular and efficient way to grow *Salvia*, since viable seeds are rare if not non-existent. You can buy cuttings from certain nurseries (see Appendix), or if you are lucky enough to have a *Salvia* enthusiast among your friends, you can take a cutting from any healthy plant. It should be a branch with four to six leaves already grown and about four inches of stem below that. By placing the stalk in water so that most of the stem below the leaves is covered, and misting to keep the humidity level up, roots will begin to appear in just a couple weeks. During this initial stage no added nutrients are needed to stimulate growth.

After the roots grow to between one-quarter to three-quarters inches, the cutting should be transplanted into soil. Longer roots are more vulnerable to damage during transplanting. Any medium-sized pot will be acceptable, as well as any potting soil. Plastic pots may be preferable to clay or terracotta pots because the soil dries out slower in plastic pots. However, one must guard against *over*-watering since plastic pots are more apt to produce root rot. Re-potting periodically is necessary since *Salvia* enjoys a lot of root space.

Every gardener has a favorite formula for his plants and asking around will yield many versions of what the "right" soil should consist of. *Salvia* doesn't grow well in heavy soils or clay-rich soils, so by steering away from those mixtures, the amateur cultivator should be fine. In the book, *The Salvia Divinorum Grower's Guide*[1], the following mixture is recommended for optimum growth:

- 1 part aged grass cuttings
- 1 part compost
- 1 part coarse sand
- 2 parts aged steer manure
- 3 parts rich soil

Other people suggest using mixtures containing parts of perlite, vermiculite, black peat and organic nutrients. In the Sierra Mazateca, the soil is rich with organic material which causes the soil to be slightly acidic. The recommended optimum soil pH is between 6.1 and 6.6. By trying different mixtures, it is possible to reproduce the indigenous growing conditions for *Salvia* to thrive.

Salvia can grow well outside under the proper conditions: shade and humidity, with partial sunlight. During the summer the growth will be the fastest and as temperatures drop and daylight hours fade, the growth will slow down. It is possible

---

[1] Sociedad Para La Preservación De Las Plantas Del Misterio, (1998) *The Salvia Divinorum Growers Guide*, Spectral Mindustries, p. 26-27.

to keep the plants indoors and use grow lights, although this will require more vigilant attention and watering as the plants can dry out quickly. Fluorescent bulbs can be used rather than fancy grow lights, which are more expensive, but, again, it is all about each gardener's personal preference. Sodium or Halide lights can also be used on *Salvia* but these are especially strong and special care will need to be given to make sure the plant does not dry out.

Salvia does not fall heavily victim to many pests but there are some to look out for. Aphids and whiteflies seem to be the most common. These pests can be combated by spraying a solution of water, castille soap and rubbing alcohol on the leaves. This is a non-toxic combination and will not harm the plant. By being attentive to *Salvia*, the sensitive gardener will notice the first signs of a pest invasion (little eggs on the underside of the leaves, or leaves that have begun to curl on the edges) and will be able to combat the pests before any serious damage is done.

Chapter Four
The Chemistry

Salvia divinorum is the only known hallucinogenic plant whose active principal is a diterpene rather than an alkaloid. Alfredo Ortega first isolated the active compound, *Salvinorin A*, while he was performing systematic tests within the *Salvia* family. He did not test the compound for its psychoactive ability in humans since his interest in the plant and research of *Salvia* was not related to this aspect of the plant. Leander Valdes and another group of scientists also isolated this compound and *did* test for its psychoactive potential but only tested the effects by administering the drug to mice. They were satisfied that *Salvinorin A* was indeed the active compound but failed to test its effects on humans. So, we were all left unaware of the very potent effects of this unique plant.

Daniel Siebert finally found what he was looking for during his experiments in the extraction of the active principal of *Salvia*. Siebert, interested mainly in the psychoactive effects of *ska Maria*, had been performing various tests and experiments on the plant in order to effectively isolate the *Salvinorin A* and then test its effect on humans. His previous experiences with the plant had been had by ingesting it the traditional way, by chewing a quid of the leaves, or drinking the extract. He was intrigued by the mild, unassuming effects of *Salvia* and was convinced that there must be a way to concentrate the psychoactive principle and thus intensify the experience of this powerful entheogen.

An Ortep Sterescopic drawing of Salvinorin

Quite by accident, Siebert produced a crystal of *Salvinorin A*. Thinking it was merely an inactive byproduct, he was about to scrap it and begin again when he was suddenly inspired to try it. A small dose, only 2.6mg, sent him on a whirlwind journey through the *Salvia* world. He had found the key.

Salvinorin A
($C_{23}H_{28}O_8$)

(1)

(2) R = H
(3) R = OAc

Salvia is made up of 96% *Salvinorin A*, the remaining 4% being *Salvinorin B*, a compound which seems to have no active psychotropic effects. Although identified and studied,

Salvinorin A still remains a bit of a mystery as no one has yet discovered exactly how it works on the brain. Tested against 500 known hallucinogens and their corresponding receptor sites in the brain, not one matches the unique *Salvinorin A*. *Salvia* is still the cryptic goddess and works her magic in mysterious ways, elusive even to scientists.

Recent research on *Salvia* along with various other entheogens like Ayahuasca has shown that *Salvinorin* is potentiated by certain MAOIs. Perhaps *Salvia* works in a similar manner, allowing certain neurons (like serotonin) to gather in the brain without inhibition, therefore triggering the effects that we know of today. The potential of this plant and the discovery of how it actually works could be an important contribution to society in many ways, not the least of which may be in psychiatric research.

As a technologically advanced society, we have not even come close to scratching the surface of the final, unknown frontier: our minds. Relatively little is known about how our brains work, or of all the intricate connections that exist within our central nervous system. Medically, we have made astounding leaps and bounds, but sadly, psychiatry lags behind, as the little sister no one wants to play with. But this little sister may hold the answer to so many questions and the tenuous connection between mind and body may be revealed to be much stronger than heretofore known.

The use of psychedelic substances has been studied in connection with psychiatry for many years but with many limitations. Because of the stigma attached to these consciousness-altering substances, mainstream society frowns upon the use or even the research of these important compounds. It may be for the very same reason that people are afraid of, and socially stigmatize, the mentally ill. People fear what they don't understand. People fear what they cannot see or touch. People fear their own minds because they do not comprehend the vast worlds therein. They choose to not look within for understanding. But for those of us who are not content to take in the surface of things without diving under and finding what lies beneath, entheogens provide the perfect tool for unlocking those mysteries.

By understanding how these substances work in the brain, we can understand the way our brains work naturally, how "mentally ill" people's brains may work differently and how their receptors are different from the average person's. With this knowledge, we will then understand how to develop effective treatments for some of these illnesses. Extensive research has been done in an effort to find effective treatments for depression. All of the treatment drugs that have been developed work in some way to close off or open up different receptors or neurotransmitters in our brains. The recent surge in the use of MAOI drugs proves that more people are looking to medicines, both plant and synthetic, to balance the delicate health of the most important and least-understood organ of the human body: the brain.

But one should not dismiss the power of the mind-body connection. Many believe that when the mind is healthy and clear, a healthy body naturally follows. This holistic approach to complete health is one that more and more people are embracing and it is fitting for *Salvia* to find her place among the herbal supplements and remedies widely circulating in the global marketplace today. This is not to say that *Salvia* can be popped in a pill like an herb such as St. John's Wort. *Salvia* is a sensitive plant and must be used with the greatest of care, temperance and knowledge. It seems more than possible that with additional research we may be able to discover the important healing properties of *Salvia divinorum,* not only for the mind, but for the body also.

Members of the *Salvia* family have been used throughout time as healers. It is no surprise that the Latin word *salveo* means "to be well." Sage has been used as a muscle relaxer, an agent against diarrhea, a tonic for sore throats, and a balm for flesh wounds. Most recently attention has turned to sages for their insulin-boosting quality which makes them a useful supplement in fighting diabetes. *Salvia divinorum,* though named for its divination abilities, follows its family's tradition of healing and has been used among the Mazatecs for various purposes.

Not only do the curanderos employ the help of *Salvia divinorum* in diagnosing the ills of a village member but also to make tonics, ointments, and baths for the ailing person. Also, the leaves can be chewed in small doses, much smaller than what would be necessary to induce a trance or any spiritual journey, and they will provide aid to the sick. *Salvia divinorum* has been thought to help with anemia, as it appears to relieve and rejuvenate a sickly person. She has also been used, as have her other sister sages, as a means for stopping diarrhea. On the other hand, *Salvia* can be used to induce defecation or urination, demonstrating that she is versatile in regulating the elimination functions in the body. It is hard to measure the worth of the herb, or many herbs for that matter, as a folk remedy for various ailments, although based on the curative history of the sage family it is easy to believe that the beautiful *Salvia divinorum* extends her magical healing hand beyond the realms of the mind and consciousness into the physical domain.

Chapter Five
Exploring Consciousness

The shamanic state of consciousness is one of non-ordinary reality. It is hard for many people of our Western culture and philosophy to grasp the concept of an alternate reality. Many feel that altered states of consciousness are nothing more than foolish escapes from the "real" ordered world that we experience on a day-to-day basis. Whether it is out of fear or ignorance, the vast majority of humans feel that the only reality is the one which they wake in, work in and experience through their five senses from the time that they are infants. Although religion may have ingrained the ideas of heaven or hell or other afterlife in the minds of some, generally it is thought that these places exist apart from us, on some other plane, which is only accessible to us after we die.

However, a growing number of enlightened, knowledgeable beings are realizing that these concepts may not be far removed from our everyday existence. This is something that shamans, medicine men, and other spiritual leaders have known all along. These people have known from the beginning of time that the "other" plane, the alternate reality, exists tangentially to our own waking consciousness and can be accessed in numerous ways, the most popular being through meditation and probably the most feared being through the use of psychotropic plants.

Fear of the unknown is both common and ironic, ironic because it is fear that keeps one from seeking knowledge. If one can overcome fear, then great stores of information will open up and the world that seemed dark and shadowy will be revealed to be full of light and knowledge. The cliché, which states that there is nothing to fear but fear itself, is right on target. If you remove fear from the equation there is no barrier between the self and the great unknown and everything becomes accessible and knowable. Of course, on the flip side of that theory is the fact that if there is one thing people fear as much as the unknown, it is knowledge itself. This is probably where the other cliché, "Ignorance is bliss," comes from.

These seemingly contradictory fears are actually one and the same. It is not actually the unknown that people are afraid of. It is what lies within the unknown; it is the final knowledge of what exists outside our physical bodies and our physical environment and within our own minds. Our lady *Salvia divinorum* can open up this unknown realm of our minds and reveal to us many of the mysteries thought to be locked away from our consciousness. No religion is necessary. This plant is the real thing, the journey, the experience and the beyond, all wrapped up neatly in the same package. Because this subject is many-layered, like our minds themselves, it is difficult to find the proper place to begin.

Since history is invaluable to understanding the future, it is there that we will start by exploring the use of *Salvia* as a divination tool by the shamans of the Mazatec culture. As discussed earlier, the curanderos of the Mazatecs used several plants in their ceremonial rituals. Each initiate into the shamanic tradition starts by exploring first the power of *Salvia*, then moving on to the other levels with morning glory seeds and the mushrooms. Each experienced curandero may use any of the plants that he or she deems appropriate for their divination rites and curing ceremonies. Some may have a special affinity to the mushrooms, as Maria Sabina did, but others may find that they favor a different ally. Don Alejandro, who helped Valdes and Diaz, felt that the mushrooms were too intense and if taken too often or in too great of a quantity had the potential to make one crazy. He preferred the gentle teachings of *ska Maria Pastora* to the whirlwind of the magic mushrooms. He explains that the visions the mushrooms can show are often "tricky" while *la Maria* is more straightforward.

Having an ally, a concept that always brings to mind Carlos Castaneda's *The Teachings of Don Juan*, is an important part of many shamanic cultures. The curanderos must have the power of many plants within their control but need their own personal ally as well. Plant gods and goddesses may need to be wooed a long time before they reveal their knowledge and power to the user. But once that alliance is established, the shaman will have a reliable guide to help him navigate the way through the "other" realm. As explained in Castaneda's book, to tame an ally requires patience, diligence, belief and ritual.

The rituals that accompany any use of the magic plant may be extremely elaborate but to the shaman they are a grave necessity. The plants are sacred to them and they would never partake of these spirits without first paying the proper homage and praying for guidance. It is through these rituals that the plant will cooperate and provide the answers to the questions of the shaman. If a person blindly eats, smokes, drinks the essence of one of these plants with no ritual, no plan and no question, they may anger the gods within and the visions that come forth may be pure terror. This leads to the ever-important "set and setting."

Set and setting refers to the way one approaches the journey of plant ecstasy. The "set" is the participant and his or her beliefs and perception. The "setting" is how one begins the journey, the place from which one starts, and the ritual, which precipitates the journey. The participant's mind-set and surroundings play an integral part in the journey. If one approaches it in a way that is not pure of heart, but with sinister intentions or with no real intention at all, the results may be stupefying. The Mazatecs, as well as all shamanic cultures, take this concept very seriously and work hard to attain an almost perfect set and setting through which they operate.

In addition to ritual preparation of the plant, which includes the separation of pairs of leaves, the grinding or chewing of those leaves, the burning of copal incense, and the prayers and incantations, which begin each ceremony, the curanderos also require darkness and silence to engage *ska Maria*. She is believed to appear only when the conditions are right and any light or noise disturbance will pull the participant back from the vision. When approached in the correct way, *la Maria* comes softly to the shaman and reveals what one needs to know — whether it be the location of a lost object or the cause of some illness. It requires knowledge, patience and practice to be able to interpret the visions of *Salvia* and the other plant gods.

It takes many years of learning to become a successful curandero and although the lessons of the plants are necessary on this path to knowledge, they are not the only requirements. One cannot ingest the plants and hope to instantly become a shaman, but one can hope to grow in enlightenment.

Having explored the traditions and history of the use of *Salvia*, we can now turn our attention to the way she might be used today. What benefits can we, in our technologically advanced, though somewhat soul-devoid, Western society, gain through the lessons of the great teacher: *ska Maria Pastora*?

The potential of *Salvia divinorum* is unlimited, not only as a possible physical curative aid, but also as a tool for broadening our minds and consciousness. She can be an unparalleled ally in this respect. But how? How can we approach this plant in a way that is advantageous without the benefit of the sociological background of the traditional shamans? The answers are easy for some — discipline and knowledge. By reading this book, you have taken the first crucial step on the path of learning.

It is important to understand how these plant allies work. Since it is unknown how *Salvia divinorum* affects the brain, we can only describe the physical effects and speculate on the rest. *Salvia* is unlike any other entheogen. It can not be compared to LSD, mescaline or even Cannabis. She is completely unique. *Salvia* seems to hold up a mirror before us and reflects the centuries that are contained in our countenances. In this way she is not unlike other psychedelic substances that are able to bring us the sense of unity with all time, space, and objects. But these are more psychological effects. The physical effects of *Salvia* are fairly mild. There is no hallucinogenic rush like that which comes from LSD, or DMT, but it is unlike the "stoning" of Cannabis either. *Salvia* creates a feeling of relaxation and a calming of the body. Some people experience a feeling of raised body temperature which can result in profuse sweating. Others become chilled. A prickling sensation can be felt all over the skin, something akin to "pins and needles" or the numbing tingle of an approaching anesthetic. This is not usually too uncomfortable, although some people don't like the creeping feeling. *Salvia* may also cause lightheadedness or dizziness, which is a good reason to be sitting comfortably or lying down while tripping. Occasional nausea was reported in accounts of people who had chewed the leaves but this is more from the bitter taste of the liquid and the gag reflex of trying to swallow a bundle of leaves than it is from the effect of *Salvia* on the stomach.

For the most part, the physical effects of the plant are as varied as the psychological effects, visiting each person in a unique way. But all people agree that the physical effects of *Salvia* are mild, short-lived and not unpleasant. There is no "crashing" when the experience is over and no hangover the next day. The entire *Salvia* experience, when it is smoked, usually lasts less than fifteen minutes with a complete return to "normal" within an hour.

There has never been a documented case of an overdose of *Salvia*. She is a non-toxic plant although obviously anything can be toxic to the body if one takes enough of it. However, she is like Cannabis in that you would have to eat/drink/smoke boatloads of the plant in order to ever reach a toxic quantity. On the other hand, *Salvinorin* is the most potent naturally occurring hallucinogen known today and there could be a danger of taking too much of this pure substance. An easy way to avoid this is by using only 6x or 5x leaf extract purchased from a reputable company such as those listed in the back of this book and by avoiding the pure substance (pure *salvinorin* A or B extract) altogether. *Salvia* sublingual tablets are now on the market and may be the most desirable method to ingest *Salvia* for those who are looking for a more subtle experience. (See the sources section in "Appendix" for *Salvia* sources.) Remember always, it is key to start off incrementally, taking small doses until one achieves the desired effect. Daniel Siebert in his initial *Salvinorin* journey only ingested 2.6

grams of *Salvinorin* and it was enough to send him spiraling into a chasm of hallucinogenic fury. Any careful explorer should have no trouble in controlling the amount of material needed to have a comfortable journey.

Since everyone's mind is different, it is impossible to say how *Salvia* will approach any individual. However there does seem to be a pattern of recognizable themes that run through the *Salvia* experience. Siebert describes them in this way:

1. Becoming objects (yellow, plaid French fries, fresh paint on a drawer, a pant leg, a Ferris Wheel, etc.).
2. Visions of various two-dimensional surfaces, films and membranes.
3. Revisiting places from the past, especially child-hood.
4. Loss of the body and/or identity.
5. Various sensations of motion, or of being pulled or twisted by forces of some kind.
6. Uncontrollable hysterical laughter.
7. Overlapping realities. The perception that one is in several locations at once.[1]

There have also been numerous reports of feeling a presence during the journey. Some people feel this is *la Maria* herself, others find that it may be an other worldly presence of a sort they cannot put their fingers on, but there is a definite sensation of being watched or guided or spoken to (even without audible words). This can be a disquieting feeling for many, although others seek out this very experience. It is a select few who feel that they have seen and interacted with the goddess, but it is a matchless encounter.

---

[1] Siebert, Daniel J., (1994) "Salvia divinorum and Salvinorin A: new pharmacologic findings," *Journal of Ethnopharmacology*, 43, p. 55.

"The Ally: she can be shy. Sometimes she has to get to know you for a while, before she will come out and say hello. But once she appears, are there any who are more direct?"[2]

Once a person has made the breakthrough, one will either be intrigued or terrified. The reaction will be almost directly correspondent to the state of mind of the participant but sometimes even those who feel prepared and who have the best intentions are not ready for the world into which *Salvia* will transport them.

Salvia is an excellent tool for exploring the inner reaches of the mind. She will not report back falsely what she finds there. As discussed before, the brain holds many mysteries and traditional psychoanalysis, pharmacological studies, and psychiatric practices only begin to scratch the surface of the almost-unlimited power of our minds. By being proactive and taking the matter of our psychological exploration into our own hands, we will not only be able to come to a serene understanding of ourselves but will also be able to add to the uplifting of humanity and the overall consciousness of the world that surrounds us. But to even approach this task, one must be free of fear and eager to follow wherever the plant teacher chooses to lead, whether or not it seems helpful or appropriate. The journey into the unknown is always going to be on a winding path with unforeseen twists and shadowy passages, but it ultimately leads to amazing vistas of truth. The key is to be receptive to all of the parts of the journey and only then will the experience be rewarding. Knowledge, both of oneself or of the world, is never a destination. It is always the journey.

So, in order to reach past the mundane experiences of our day-to-day life and reach new plateaus of insight, we must

---

[2] Pendell, Dale, (1995) *Pharmako/poeia: Plant Powers, Poisons, and Herbcraft*, Mercury House, San Francisco.

embark on an adventure into the "other" realm, the alternate reality, the shamanic landscape. This alternative reality is a reality directed within us, an inner consciousness that links everyone together throughout space and time, at all points connecting. It is not a dimension outside of our three-dimensional lives, but accessed inside, in our virtually unexplored minds. In the brain/mind lies the pathway to another world and psychotropic plants can be used to unlock the gate that guards it. Boundaries, both physical and mentally conditioned by society, keep us from reaching too deeply inside our brains for fear of what we might find.

This is exactly why entheogenic substances like *Salvia divinorum* can be so powerful and transformative, because they dissolve boundaries. If one is diligent and earnest and curious enough to push and bend those boundaries, he may be successful in breaking through to this alternate reality. At the very least, he will gain a new perspective. *Salvia*, although temperamental like all divine women, can be a guide on this journey.

The best way to begin the exploration is by using small doses of *Salvia* for meditation. There is a definite threshold between a small amount, which should put one into a calm, non-distracted state of mind perfect for guided meditation, and a dose that will make one lose control over the experience and put one at the mercy of la dame *Salvia*.

About one gram or less of dried *Salvia divinorum* leaf should be sufficient to begin a meditative journey. Meditation is an invaluable tool, not only for personal insight, but also for allowing the brain to take a respite from the constant barrage of information it must deal with every waking moment. The brain needs this rest in order to function with clarity and to "cleanse the doors of perception." Although the aforemen-

tioned cleansing is usually thought to reference only the experience of a hallucinogenically induced trance, it can also be
initiated through meditation, detoxification, and/or fasting.

There is currently research underway sponsored by MAPS,
the Multidisciplinary Association for Psychedelic Studies, to
evaluate *Salvia divinorum* as a tool for meditation work. The
participants are divided into three groups, two receiving different doses of the plant and one group receiving a placebo.
The initial results of the research have been positive and the
experiments are ongoing.

Aside from meditation, *Salvia* can be helpful with other
forms of self-exploration, as long as one is willing to see what
is truly inside. *Salvia* pulls no punches. She can arrive, almost
without warning, and whisk one off into a surreal hyperspace
filled with images either fanciful or horrifying. To attempt to
describe a typical experience is almost self-defeating. There is
nothing typical about *Salvia*. One can only get an idea of her
modus operandi by listening to others' meetings with her.

"It felt that when I smoked the *Salvinorin* I had remembered
who I was. I remembered I was consciousness, not a body,
and, as consciousness, I had access to unlimited realms. Another perception of what took place is that the 'I' that smoked
the *Salvinorin* dissolved into infinity and a different, but
similar, entity jumped out of infinity into the body that was
lying on the bed. This seemed to be an explanation for my
body's fear. My body knew it was going to be losing the
'spirit' which had been inhabiting it, and was going to have a
new spirit come inside."[3]

---

[3] Turner, D.M., (1996) *Salvinorin: The Psychedelic Essence of Salvia
Divinorum*, Panther Press.

A common internal perception that comes from smoking *Salvia* is the dissolution of identity boundaries. There becomes no more body, but only consciousness that may take many forms. This can be a marvelous and an almost epiphanic moment for some, in the way that it reinforces the idea that we are all part of a larger unity of consciousness that extends from our minds or souls. It can also be an intensely uncomfortable feeling when one feels the loss of "being human" and instead finds himself inhabiting some other object. This has the possibility of being a pleasant sensation (if a little strange) such as an explorer who enjoyed becoming a tree. It also has the ability of being quite disturbing, as described here by D.M. Turner:

"I was not a person, nor did I remember ever having been a person, or taken any drug... I was perceiving everything as though I was an exterior wall of a house. I soon realized that I was 'glued' to this particular existence as the side of a house. I had become something inanimate and material, yet I was aware of life around me, and knew that I had recently been a particular human being... I tried to return to my previous human identity and found that I was unable to do so. I felt that I was stuck for eternity as the side of this house, and an acute sense of fear and terror began to develop. I did not feel particularly uncomfortable, only somewhat when I attempted to return to my human identity and found myself unable to do so. I felt perturbed at whoever gave me this bizarre psychedelic. Why would someone give me a substance which would leave me eternally existing as the side of a house?"[4]

This dissolution of identity and distortion of time and place is the magical, yet slightly frightening, power of *Salvia*. The entire time-space continuum, which we exist in day to day, is

---

[4] *Ibid.*

completely rearranged. One may feel eternally stuck to the side of a house and yet in "real" time only ten minutes have elapsed. Another aspect of this time distortion is the ability to seemingly move about in points of time.

Terrence McKenna, psychonaut extraordinaire, speculated that time travel might not be in the strange time machines of science fiction but rather an inner ability to access all points of infinity within our own minds.

Daniel Siebert, who is a *Salvia* expert, mentions repeatedly, in his lectures and writings, his experiences in traveling to different moments of his past and in accessing places from his childhood memories. In the description of his first intense experience with *Salvinorin*, he explains how he repeatedly seemed to end up in different people's living rooms, one being his maternal grandparents', furnished as it was when he was a child. He says, "Some of these places were from my childhood and some were from my more recent past. In this state all the points of time in my personal history coexisted. One did not precede the next. Apparently, had I so willed it, I could return to any point in my life and really be there, because it was actually happening right now."[5]

Reports of experiences like these reinforce the shamanic world belief of all points of time and space coexisting. This makes it possible, with proper tools like *Salvia*, for us to maneuver, not only through our minds, but through different arenas of space and time both in our natural reality and the "alternative" reality of the gods. Now some might find this idea overblown or simply ludicrous, the stuff of children's tales

---

[5] *Ibid.*

and science fiction. But one encounter with our lady *Salvia* should make believers of them all.

The *Salvia* experience is a lot like a dream. We find imagery we recognize from our waking lives just slightly twisted into a sometimes confusing, sometimes illuminating, way of thinking. There are many theories as to what produces dreams. Some believe that it is excess sensory input unprocessed during the day that the brain stores away to be dealt with during our dream states at night. Others believe that dreams are messages and symbols from our subconscious. Still others think that dreams are nothing but the fractal light images produced by the REM cycle and have no meaning other than what our over-active, analytical minds superimpose upon them. In any case, dreaming is an important brain process that has only begun to be thoroughly researched and has not even begun to be fully understood.

There is a faction of people who are involved in exploring the dream consciousness and who are successful at controlling their own dreams. This process, lucid or conscious dreaming, may be another meaningful step in understanding the mysterious realms of our brain. It is hypothesized that a person is able to confront the images in their dreams and find out from the source what information is to be taken away from the experience. People successful in lucid dreaming find that they can take care of important issues during their sleep state, which leaves their brain uncluttered to take on the tasks of everyday living during waking hours. People have reported instances of being able to go back and right old wrongs or to heal sources of pain from the past. Is this another case of time travel within the mind? Or is it perhaps being able to transport oneself to another time and place in this dimension or another? Maybe it is possible that our dream world is actually that "alternate" reality we have been seeking. If so, the world we journey to with *Salvia* is the same world we encounter in our dreams.

To have a conscious dream one must exercise a lot of control. This takes time and discipline, but the results are astounding. One finds oneself asleep but keenly aware of what is taking place. One is then able to "take over" the dream, to maneuver through the new realm and accomplish whatever goals are intended. As with *Salvia* it is a good idea to have a clearly defined intention when taking on a conscious dream. This will greatly enhance the experience. *Salvia* may be able to help in the conscious dreaming process in much the same way it is helpful in meditation. Small doses may heighten brain sensitivity to an appropriate level so that a conscious dream is possible. Too much *Salvia* will cause the user to lose the control necessary to successfully navigate the experience.

However, even larger doses of *Salvia* can be useful in exploring the dream world of alternate reality. If the participant allows *Salvia* to lead the way and gives her the control over the experience, he may find that *Salvia* has a good handle on what needs to be learned. It is just a matter of being receptive to whatever the plant goddess wishes to teach us, even if we aren't sure we really want to know. This can be a danger, especially with *Salvia*. The inner thoughts, fears, desires, personalities, and inclinations of our minds are opened for inspection and it might not always be a pretty sight. In fact it is rarely what we expect but it is usually imperative for the soul, on its way to enlightenment, to confront every part of the mind, even the parts one wishes to keep locked away from the world. But *Salvia* holds the key to all those locks and is not afraid to use them.

Thousands, if not millions, of people engage in psychotherapy of some sort every year. People are anxious to find out what makes them tick, what drives them, what secret barriers keep them from achieving their ultimate actualization.

Salvia, the Diviner's Sage, the Seer's Sage, could be an invaluable asset to psychiatric treatment, not only by helping reveal how the brain works while taking *Salvinorin* (as discussed earlier), but also by enhancing the self-exploration which is engaged in while undergoing therapy. The *Salvia* experience has the potential to provide profound insight into the trappings of one's mind, especially when taken under the proper setting and, in this case, with the proper guidance. A knowledgeable, holistic therapist or healer would be able to employ *Salvia* to great ends by guiding their patient through the experience and helping them to make sense of the feelings and imagery that accompany the *Salvia* trance.

Using psychedelic plants and drugs in psychiatry has long been a controversial topic. Timothy Leary tried to show the world the benefits of LSD therapy and, unfortunately, succeeded only in turning more people against it. Now most psychedelics are controlled substances and research into their possible medical or psychiatric benefits is outlawed.

Salvia divinorum is not a controlled substance, however. This gives our little plant ally a chance at becoming what the other psychedelics can't: a useful, medico-psycho-therapeutic aid for living.

How has *Salvia* avoided the condemning powers-that-be? Until recently the psychoactive principal *Salvinorin* had yet to be discovered. Therefore, any effects reported to the general public were based on speculation and hearsay. Many scientists didn't even believe that the plant held any real hallucinogenic properties and that the chronicled effects of *Salvia* were nothing more than a placebo effect. Now, that *Salvinorin A* has been isolated and has proven its entheogenic power beyond a shadow of a doubt, many people wonder how long it will be before Big Brother puts an end to *Salvia*'s freedom. But *Salvia* is different in so many ways from her illegal, psychoactive comrades.

First of all, *Salvia* can not really be used as a recreational drug. The effects vary from a mild, relaxing, non-hallucinogenic state to an intense, self-revealing, psychedelic whirlwind. Neither of these two extremes is conducive to overuse or abuse. For those wishing to use a drug to escape, *Salvia* is not going to be their choice. If anything, *Salvia* will hold you captive in whatever mental state you might be trying to escape. The sensory side effects of *Salvia* are pleasant, but not so euphoric that people would seek out the experience when there are other more immediate, and more sensual, effects to be had by some other drugs.

Salvia is an introspective drug; she is a thinking, feeling drug. She can be a life-changing drug but only to those sensitive people who are willing to devote the time, energy, and discipline required to get to know and understand her. *Salvia* will never be a drug pushed on the street. She will never be whispered in the ear of concert-goers. A plant that is most effective when taken alone in a darkened, quiet place is not destined to become appealing to the masses.

Salvia is simply not a party drug, but a tool for those interested in expanding their consciousness. Many who try *Salvia* find that they are scared of her and will not go back. It is the fear of knowledge that will keep the unenlightened away and the thrill of knowledge that will keep the learned, responsible explorers coming back for more.

Another reason why *Salvia* may be able to escape the clutches of the law is because of its relative obscurity. Those who do know of the plant, *Salvia divinorum,* and who know of the treasure that is buried in her leaves are not anxious for her to be exploited. Those who feel a natural affinity for *Salvia* also feel the natural urge to protect her. Information about her is shared within several communities of sensitive souls who are interested only in helping others attain a higher consciousness. Despite the volume of material available on the Internet, *Salvia* is still not a well-known, household name even among members of the counter-culture. And many *Salvia* devotees would prefer to keep it that way.

So why write a book extolling the virtues of *ska Maria Pastora?* Because she is too beautiful to keep out of the light forever. Because there are millions of people out there, just like you, who can benefit from her teachings. And because knowledge is power. As long as we can educate those willing to learn, and allow the facts of the history and growth of *Salvia divinorum* be known before her name is polluted with fallacies in mainstream society, then we can protect *Salvia* from the danger that ultimately springs from ignorance.

Chapter Six
Reflections

Since all experiences with *Salvia* are subjective and best described by the individuals who experience them, this section is devoted to reports of individual research and exploration of the Diviner's Sage. All names have been changed to protect the identity of the psychonauts.

"I decided to try smoking *Salvia* out of a pipe-bowl even though I had been told this was an ineffective way. I wasn't really anxious to have a mind-blowing, psychedelic experience so I figured that this would be the best way to avoid inhaling too much. I did have to smoke at least four or five bowls full before I got the desired effect. After the first three bowls, I felt a bit lightheaded from all the inhaling but I didn't get the sense that anything out of the ordinary was happening. After at least a half an hour I smoked another two bowls and began to feel as if I was drifting off... kind of away from my body. I could feel the delicate balance between consensus reality and the otherworldly feeling of a trip coming on. I have taken enough psychedelics in my time to know when I've reached the threshold. I felt good, not uneasy or anything, but I knew I didn't want to go any further. I allowed myself to empty my mind and see into myself and I was able to hold this meditative state for about a half an hour or so. Once my downstairs neighbors came home, the noise distracted me and I was snapped fully back into the present reality. It was a quite peaceful experience and I could see how *Salvia* could be useful in meditation as long as you don't take too much. I was bordering on too much but I felt like I could still control it. Maybe after a few more meditative sessions I will attempt to 'meet' *ska Maria* as I have heard others talk about but I know I am not ready just yet..." — *Marcus*

"The house was actually quiet for once so I thought it would be a good time to smoke *Salvia*. Even though I had been warned not to take it alone, I thought that I was responsible enough to take care of myself so I locked the doors and gave it a shot. What a mistake! I could feel the approach of the drug after only about 2 grams worth. The other times I had tried *Salvia* I had taken more, and anyway the steady buzz I had come to expect arrived much earlier than usual. The buzz in my ear became more of a full body vibration that was slightly uncomfortable. At the periphery of my sight I could see the edges of my perception beginning to curl inward. It was as if I was looking at a giant picture that was pasted on a background of nothingness and all of reality was beginning to fold in on itself leaving nothing behind. For a half a moment I thought the visual was pretty cool but then I became scared and felt like I was going to be folded in on as well. The next thing I knew I was sitting on my bathroom floor with my head in my hands like I was hiding. Hiding from the drug?! I don't know what I was thinking... but when I finally looked around me and saw that my vision was whole and not curling at the edges I was able to calm down a bit. Then I heard whispering which freaked me out a bit since I thought I was alone but then I had the distinct sense that I was not alone. In the corner of my eye

I could see a figure but every time I moved my head to look at it, it disappeared. I chased my tail like this for what seemed like forever, eventually left the bathroom and began looking in corners for the mysterious figure. When I finally gave up I laid myself out on the bed and closed my eyes. I was able to attain the feeling of floating that I love so much and found myself wishing that I hadn't wasted my experience hiding in the bathroom. That's when I knew that reality was creeping back in. I was exhausted and felt like I had been through a weeklong ordeal. When I looked at the clock I saw that only twelve minutes had passed. I think I will always have a sitter from now on." — *Melissa*

"I knew it was coming, I could feel it but I still wasn't really sure what to expect, and then Bam! My eyesight seemed to go out and all I could see was this tiny pinhole in the center of the darkness and then just as quick it was like I was seeing through the hole, you know like that movie with the tunnel, you know, with the rabbits? Alice and Wonderland, right, and then I was in the tunnel and it felt like I was getting sucked into a vacuum and Kelly was there (the sitter) and I was holding her hand so we wouldn't both get sucked in and I could see the door, a tiny door, and I had my hand on it but it wouldn't open and I was scared that we were both going to get sucked away, and I could see Kelly but she kept getting further and further away and then Billy walked in and I had a dose of what was really happening and the vision disappeared and I realized I was OK." — *Christine*

"I could see that Christine was upset and kind of panicking. Her eyes were really wide and she was reaching out to the table and grabbing it as if to hold on or keep her bearings or something. She asked me if she was OK and I said yes and she said, 'You're with me' and I said 'Yes, I'm with you,' but then she started saying she was scared and she was holding my hand really tight. So, I squeezed her hand and told her it was going to be all right, that it would all be over soon. She kept grasping at the table. After Billy came into the room, she seemed to calm down and then she just started laughing hysterically. When the trip was finally over and she told us what she saw I was amazed. My experiences have never been like that!" — *Kelly*

"I had been smoking Marijuana with some friends when someone brought out the *Salvia*. I hadn't ever taken it but I was really curious. After about two bowls full I felt like I was snapped into another world. Everything looked like a photo negative of itself. I had this idea that I had entered the flip side and those words kept running through my mind. Then suddenly, I was lying on my back and there was green, green, green grass all around me and it was really soft and I felt like I was a part of it. My friends told me I was rubbing my body all over the carpet like I was a dog. But I just had this wonderful feeling like I was a part of the earth and it was so peaceful and I had no concept of time nor did I really care..." — *Roger*

"After taking a couple of hits and feeling nothing I was almost convinced I was immune. Then I figured another hit wouldn't kill me. I was right. I began to laugh; everything was suddenly uncontrollably funny. John started asking me questions like what was so funny and as I tried to answer him it looked like he was becoming a brick wall. One by one these white bricks began to fill in my vision, I could still kind of see John's face but the whole thing was kind of creepy and suddenly I wasn't laughing anymore." — *Greg*

"I took more than I probably should have, probably close to 3 grams, and I have never had a more profound experience in my life. I found myself in a forest surrounded by all of these intricate branches. At first I couldn't tear my eyes away from them, the geometric patterns were so beautiful. But then I had the definite sense of a presence and I felt like I was being led away deeper into this forest. I couldn't see who I was following but I knew I was following someone... *ska Maria* possibly... but definitely someone or something, I don't know, I just felt compelled. But then my vision got dark and it seemed I was at a crossroads and I was saying that I didn't want to go on but I had to. When I realized I had no choice I just gave myself over to the experience and found myself hurtling through space; my body was twisting and turning. It was crazy. Then I landed and felt as if my body was sinking into the ground. I was in reality lying on my bed and thought I had been the entire time but it is possible that I got up and was walking around. Anyway, as I sank into the ground I noticed little falling stars in my vision all different brightly colored specks falling through the darkness. But then I felt the tingling sensation and it was like a million little needles pricking me, not painful really, just mildly annoying and I saw that the brightly colored stars had begun to collect over me as if they were little grains of sand. I was being buried alive but I didn't care. I just watched the colored sand cover me and had the vague feeling that this wasn't the worst way to go. Then my dog jumped up on the bed and I could feel him but it felt like he was way above me on the mattress and I was just feeling the vibrations from underneath. This began to bring me out of the vision and I struggled to get back to the real plane where I knew my dog was. After I attained a normal sense of self, I had this overwhelming feeling of sadness. I missed the *Salvia* world." — *James*

All of the above-recorded reports are somewhat typical of the *Salvia* experience, even though they are all very different. The sense of leaving one's body or of feeling one's body in motion, whether it be flying, floating, sinking or hurtling through space, are all common with *Salvia*. Even though each experience is unique there are common threads that run through the trips. How the trip will go depends heavily upon set and setting and the cultural and societal influences that affect our perceptions. In this context, it is easy to see how a shaman may ingest *Salvia* and be able to divine the root of an illness through communicating with the gods and how someone from our Western culture would find *Salvia* an interesting experience of light and pattern but would have no access to an unfathomable alternate reality. We are only able to perceive what we know and our life and conscious reality is made up of these perceptions.

Salvia may be able to expand one's mind but only if one believes there is something other than the reality one breathes every day. A participant in the *Salvia* experience must be receptive to an alternative way of thinking.

Our cultural constructs make up so much of our thought patterns and we barely recognize it. The ideas of our culture become ingrained in us from an early age and in our ethnocentrism we take for granted that this is just the way things are. Unfortunately, this could be a danger to *Salvia*. Because so many people believe that all psychedelic plants are the same and that all psychedelics are dangerous, *Salvia* may get a bad reputation just by being a unique member of an entheogenic group. In shamanic cultures, these plants are holy and sacred. They are an integral part of a unified world of plant and animal spirits. Their culture, religion, and world philosophies hinge on the use of these sacred plants. In our culture we are taught that all psychedelic drugs are bad.

Almost all psychedelic drugs are illegal. It will be hard to change an entire culture's view on the basis of one special plant. But we can try.

It is important for those of us interested in expanding our consciousness and exploring alternative worldviews to learn from the ancient wisdom of the shamans. They understand the power of the plant gods and goddesses and know how to harness that power. They are able to enter the realm of plants like *Salvia* and bring important information back to our own dimension. By studying, learning, and exploring, we too can learn the wisdom of *Salvia* and use the wisdom for personal growth and worldly understanding.

The Dreamer's Gate

An Exercise for Reproducing the Salvia divinorum Experience

Once you have had a *Salvia divinorum* experience, it is possible to reproduce the *Salvia divinorum* experience without the use of *Salvia divinorum*. It is the space in time that is known to the shaman as "The Dreamer's Gate." When the Diviner's Sage is not in season a shaman can replicate the experience through a series of techniques.

The technique begins each time you take *Salvia divinorum* (preferably from the first time) and its success is in part attributed to anchoring certain stimuli to the experience with the substance. When the circumstance is replicated identically except for the substance the same effects can be achieved. This technique, however, requires that you have had at least three *Salvia divinorum* experiences using the same stimuli, at least one of which is a threshold experience.

Step 1
Creating a Sacred Space
Just as the shaman creates a sacred space where he administers the *Salvia* sacrament, you too must create a sacred space. Do whatever is meaningful to you. Make the space sa-

cred to you. Notice everything that is around you and duplicate it each time before you have the experience.

Step 2
Light

Turn off all of the lights and have only a single candle burning. Light it thoughtfully with a match. Notice the flicker of the candle each time before the experience. Do not light candles during the next few weeks or months, to make it a specific anchor for this experience.

Step 3
Sound

(This is an optional stimulus that may be omitted as some people prefer silence.) Select a CD or tape that is appropriate and play this music before during and after the experience. Do not play this music at any other time, except when having a *Salvia divinorum* experience. A good CD for this purpose is the Metronome CD which is listed in the sources section of "Appendix".

Step 4
Smell

Lighting a particular incense, burning sage or using a specific essential oil also proves quite useful. Once again, you should not use this scent at any other time, only when having a *Salvia* experience.

Step 5
The Meditation

A special mantra, prayer or even a thought can be used. It does not have to be anything in particular, so long as it is something that is special and meaningful to you. It is important that it is exactly the same each time. It is crucial to enter into a meditative trance state prior to taking the substance. There are many good books on meditation and trance states.

Step 6
The Gate

Since there is no telling what the subconscious notices and what it doesn't, really try hard not to forget any detail about your experience. Take painstaking care to duplicate the experience identically each time. Notice everything. Every little detail counts and is important.

When you are ready to try to enter the Dreamer's Gate without the use of any substance then all you have to do is replicate the circumstance. Take your time and do everything as if you were taking the substance. Follow the ritual you have laid out. Play your music and burn your incense. Repeat your sacred words. But this time instead of taking the substance, close your eyes and visualize your self having taken it. See the smoke rise up through your body. Feel the feelings you felt when you first took it. If at first you notice only mild effects, try again until you achieve the desired effects.

Sometimes for some people it may take several attempts and several *Salvia divinorum* experiences before they can duplicate it without the substance. If you keep trying however, sooner or later it will happen. It may begin in a dream or it may begin in a meditation and then turn into a dream. Nevertheless, you will find yourself transported to a bridge between this world and the other. You will be at the Dreamer's Gate.

Appendix

Additional References

Castaneda, Carlos, *The Teachings of Don Juan*: *A Yaqui Way of Knowledge,* 1998, University of California Press.

DeKorne, Jim, *Psychedelic Shamanism: The Cultivation, Preparation and Shamanic Use of Psychotropic Plants*, 1994, Breakout Productions.

Ecstacy: Journal of Divine Experience, Issue #2, The Center For Sacred Plant Research.

Schultes, Richard Evans, and Albert Hofmann, *Plants of the Gods*, 1992, Healing Arts Press.

Salvia Divinorum Home Page With Comprehensive Links (the author's Web page): www.divining ecstasy.com

Salvia Divinorum Sources and Suppliers

Salvia Divinorum Leaf, Extract, Tablets, Videos, CD ROMS, and many other items. Metronome CD by Stuart

Wilde mentioned on page 62 is available for $19.99 from the Temple of Ecstacy.
Shamanic Transformations: www.templeofecstacy.com

Temple of Ecstacy Corporation
PO Box 16442
Beverly Hills, CA 90209-2442
1-800-365-0000

Vaporizers and other smokeless systems: air-12.com.

Salvia Divinorum Plants

Companion Plants
7247 N. Coolville Ridge Rd.
Athens, OH 45701

Logee's Greenhouses, Ltd.
141 North Street
Danielson, CT 06239-1939

Native Habitat Ethnobotanicals
PO Box 644023
Vero Beach, FL 32964-4023

Botanic Arts (Excellent Hydroponic Salvia)
Postbus 81
3140 AB Maassluis-NL
Holland

Gnostic Garden
PO Box 242
Newcastle NE99 1ED
England

For additional nurseries (inside and outside the US) please check with the author's Web site: www.diviningecstasy.com for an updated list.

You Will Also Want to Read:

❑ **85182 PSYCHEDELIC SHAMANISM: The Cultivation, Preparation and Shamanic Use of Psychotropic Plants,** *by Jim DeKorne.* From the author of *Hydroponic Hot House* comes the boldest exploration of psychedelic plants since Terence McKenna's *Food of the Gods.* DeKorne is a "psychonaut" exploring the "imaginal realms" through personal experimentation and scholarly research. He guides the reader through the history and lore of psychotropic plants, with advice on how to handle the eerie "entities" one encounters in "hyperspace." Plants and combinations covered include: Belladonna Alkaloids; D-Lysergic Acid Amide; Mescaline; Ayahuasca; Smokable DMT from Plants; Psilocybin; and more. *1994, 8½ x 11, 163 pp, illustrated, indexed, soft cover.* **$19.95**

❑ **85186 OPIUM FOR THE MASSES: A Practical Guide to Growing Poppies and Making Opium,** *by Jim Hogshire.* Everything you ever wanted to know about the beloved poppy and its amazing properties, including: What does the opium high feel like?; The stunning similarities between opium and your body's natural endorphins; Morphine and its derivatives; How to grow opium poppies; Sources for fertile poppy seeds; And much more! Also includes rare photographs and detailed illustrations. *1994, 5½ x 8½, 112 pp, illustrated, indexed, soft cover.* **$14.95**

❑ **85346 HERBS OF THE NORTHERN SHAMAN, A Guide to Mind-Altering Plants of the Northern Hemisphere,** *by Steve Andrews.* This book describes in clear, understandable terms the plants and fungi, their active constituents, the dosages, and their effects on the human mind and body. Whether you are an explorer of alternative realities or a botany buff and consummate student this book is for you. *2000, 8½ x 11, 116 pp, illustrated, indexed, soft cover.* **$14.95**

❑ **85276 INVISIBLE MARIJUANA AND PSYCHEDELIC MUSHROOM GARDENS,** *by Robert Bunch.* This book is unlike other "grow" books, in that the emphasis is on how to keep your garden hidden. This book reveals the "High in the Sky" system, which the author has found to be foolproof! The author says, "People are going to grow and smoke dope, that is all there is to it. I am just providing an easier way to grow marijuana that also has the benefit of being risk-free. If you have an invisible marijuana garden, no one can see it. And as you well know, if there is no witness, there is no crime." *Sold for informational purposes only. 1998, 8½ x 11, 150 pp, illustrated, soft cover.* **$17.95**

❑ **14133 THE HYDROPONIC HOT HOUSE, Low-Cost, High-Yield Greenhouse Gardening, *by James B. DeKorne*.** An illustrated guide to alternative-energy greenhouse gardening. Includes directions for building several different greenhouses; practical advice on harnessing solar energy; and many hard-earned suggestions for increasing plant yield. This is the first easy-to-use guide to home hydroponics. This hard-core working manual for the serious gardener is fully illustrated with diagrams, charts, and photographs. *1992, 5½ x 8½, 178 pp, illustrated, indexed, soft cover.* **$16.95**

❑ **85203 STONED FREE, How to Get High Without Drugs, *by Patrick Wells with Douglas Rushkoff*.** Now you can just say "NO!" to drugs… and get high anyway! This book enumerates many drugless consciousness-altering techniques, both timeless and recent in origin, that anyone can make use of. Meditation, breathing techniques, high-tech highs, sleep and dream manipulation, and numerous other methods are examined in detail. Avoid incarceration, save money, and skip the wear and tear on your body, while getting higher than a kite. *1995, 5½ x 8½, 157 pp, illustrated, soft cover.* **$14.95**

❑ **85283 ADVANCED TECHNIQUES OF CLANDESTINE PSYCHEDELIC & AMPHETAMINE MANUFACTURE, *by Uncle Fester*.** Underground America's most popular chemist shares his secrets in this volume, designed to make assorted trips accessible to the masses. The Fester Formula makes the best use of modern technology so the product is simple, clean, and best of all — hangover free. Special chapters include tips on how to get started, how to set up your lab with easily accessible materials, such as lithium from batteries and a transformer from a toy train. You'll also learn how to stay out of jail from pros who know. *Sold for informational purposes only. 1998, 5½ x 8½, 200 pp, soft cover.* **$27.95**

❑ **85102 RECREATIONAL DRUGS, *by Professor Buzz*.** The single finest book ever written on the manufacture of recreational drugs. Profusely illustrated, it covers the equipment, techniques and reagents used in the clandestine manufacture of illegal drugs. Procedures for crystallization, chromatography, distillation and reductions are given for the following types of drugs: amphetamines, hallucinogens; THC; analgesics; hypnotics, sedatives, and tranquilizers. Also includes detailed instructions for buying and making precursors. *Sold for informational purposes only. 1989, 8½ x 11, 166 pp, illustrated, soft cover.* **$21.95**

❏ **85241 PRACTICAL LSD MANUFACTURE, Revised and Expanded Second Edition**, *by Uncle Fester.* This book contains the most detailed, comprehensive and concise descriptions ever compiled of several innovative procedures for extracting LSD from natural sources, as well as stunning breakthrough in psychedelic drug preparation: a simple process for extracting the hallucinogenic substance 2,4,5-trimethoxyamphetamine (TMA-2) from the common, widely available calamus plant! Also includes tips on solvent management, cautionary notes and more. *Sold for informational purposes only. 1997, 5½ x 8½, 160 pp, illustrated, soft cover.* **$20.00**

Please send me the books I have marked below:

❏ **85182, Psychedic Shamanism, $19.95**
❏ **85186, Opium For The Masses, $14.95**
❏ **85346, Herbs of the Northern Shaman, $14.95**
❏ **85276, Invisible Marijuana and Psychedelic Mushroom Gardens, $14.95**
❏ **14133, The Hydroponic Hot House, $16.95**
❏ **85203, Stoned Free, $14.95**
❏ **85283, Advanced Techniques of Clandestine Psychedelic & Amphetamine Manufacture, $27.95**
❏ **85102, Recreational Drugs, $21.95**
❏ **85241, Practical LSD Manufacture, $20.00**
❏ **88888, 2001 Loompanics Unlimited Main Catalog, $5.00 (*Free* if you order any of the above titles)**

Loompanics Unlimited
PO Box 1197
Port Townsend, WA 98368

DE01

I have enclosed $ _____ which includes $5.95 for shipping and handling of the first $25 ordered. I have added $1 for each additional $25 ordered. Washington residents include 8.2% sales tax.

Name _____

Address_____

City/State/Zip_____

We accept Visa, Discover, and MasterCard. To place a credit card order only call **toll-free 1-800-380-2230**, 24 hours a day, 7 days a week.
Check out our Web site: **www.loompanics.com**